LOW CARB FOOD LIST FOR BEGINNERS

An easy guide to living the low carb life with 7 days easy to follow low carb nutritional plan

Snow A Ryan

Copyright

All Rights Reserved. Contents in this book may not be copied in any way or by means without written consent of the publisher, with the exclusion of brief excerpt in critical reviews and articles.

Snow A Ryan © 2021

Disclaimer

This book is expected to be a general guide to raise awareness and help people make a knowledgeable choice in their condition. The author takes no accountability for any damage or injury, be it individual or financial, due to the use or misuse of the information in this book. If you have any worries or fears after reading this book, do well to speak to a trained individual before further action

Table of content

Chapter 1 1
   Introduction 1
Chapter 2 3
   Best low carb meats, poultry's and eggs 3
Chapter 3 12
   Fish and shellfish as a low carb food 12
Chapter 4 13
   Best low carb Nut flours 13
Chapter 5 16
   Best low carb vegetables 16
Chapter 6 28
   Best low carb fruits and berries 28
Chapter 7 38
   Best low carb drinks 38
Chapter 8 42
   Low carb Nuts & Seeds 42
Chapter 9 50
   The best Alcohol to be taken when on low carb diet ... 50
Chapter 10 53
   Low carb dairy 53
Chapter 11 56
   Best low carb fats 56
Chapter 12 60
   7 days easy to follow low carb nutritional plan 60

Chapter 1

Introduction

A low-carb diet means a way to reduce the number of carbs we normally have, mostly found in sugary foods, pasta and bread. You are to eat fewer carbohydrates and a higher proportion of fat, vegetable, and protein, which plays an important role in weight loss. In low carb diet, you have to minimize your intake of sugar and starches; instead, you can eat more of natural fat, natural protein such as meat, which is an excellent source of protein, although the best is grass feed or extensive pasture-based system because it improves the nutritional value and reduces the risk of inflammation and probably reduce the risk of heart disease, as well the ratio of omega-3 and omega-6 fats is far better in grass-fed than in intensive based system, fish is also rich in protein and is an acceptable low carb food, still if possible choose oily fish, eggs as well is packed with protein, vegetables the best is the ones growing above the ground. You don't need to use special weight lose product or count your intake of calories or weigh your food to loss weight for studies show that low-carb diets help in promoting weight loss and likewise to control your blood sugar and improved health signs, never starve yourself all you need to do is to eat when hungry and stop when you are satisfied. Still, you have to plan, so you aren't tempted to eat foods not found on the list.

This low carb food list is an easy guide to help you kick start the reduction of your daily net carb intake to an average and it also contain the number of carb per 100gram of your foods, enjoy the foods from the below list of acceptable low carb vegetables, fats, protein and nuts. Below are examples of what you could eat and also 7 days easy to follow low carb nutritional plans and recipes

Chapter 2

Best low carb meats, poultry's and eggs

Beef meat

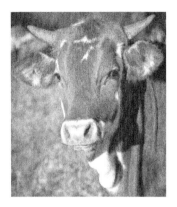

Beef is a rich source of protein, which the best is mainly produced in extensive pasture-based systems. It contains highly valuable vital nutrients facts such as- iron, zinc, selenium thiamine, riboflavin, niacin, vitamin B6, vitamin B12, vitamin D, phosphorus, magnesium, potassium and 179 calories in a 3-ounces portion. Beef as 0% carbohydrate is important in the human diet to secure a long and healthy life, without nutritional deficiencies

Chicken meat

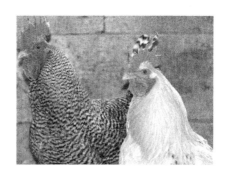

Chicken is a high source of protein and whereas low in calories and fat compared to other meats. Chicken is low in carbohydrates no matter the part you cut. That is to say, if, on a low-carb diet, it may be a healthier choice to make. Chicken as food has different parts and ways of preparation. You can alternatively eat any part such as Chicken thighs, chicken wings, chicken breast, chicken drumstick, gizzard and so on. All are acceptable low cab food. It contains 162 calories in a 3-ounces portion, and essential nutrients such as Fat, Saturated fat, Omega-3, Omega-6, Protein, Vitamin B, Vitamin B6, Vitamin B5, Vitamin B12, Vitamin B1, Vitamin B2, folate, vitamin E, vitamin K, vitamin A, selenium, phosphorus, potassium, magnesium, zinc, iron, sodium, copper, calcium, manganese, all these nutrients are important in daily human diets

Duck meat

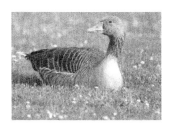

Ducks, like other poultry, are a good source of protein even as often being affiliated with a high-fat content food, it has an additional nutrient-dense than you think. It comprises mostly healthy unsaturated fat and a combination of omega-3 and omega-6, which is heart-healthy fatty acids, but still has rich meat. Duck is an excellent choice of a low carb food for it does not contain any carbohydrates, it contains 115 calories in each 3-ounce portion, and it also contains a variety of micronutrients, including iron, selenium which is a vital antioxidant that can help prevent cell damage and fight inflammation and no or a small amount of vitamin C. It contains vitamin B, B-12 is essential for nerve function, vitamin A, calcium, sodium, potassium, cobalamin magnesium is high in niacin, which plays a vital role in converting carbohydrates into glucose and metabolizing fats and proteins.

Goat meat

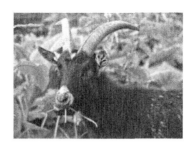

Goat meat is full of proteins, which is an important nutrient the body needs daily and contains very little cholesterol; hence, it can be consumed frequently. It has lower fat content than beef and chicken and far lesser calories, of which a 3-ounces portion of goat meat contains 122 calories, though the best is mainly produced in an extensive pasture-based system. Goat meat does not contain any carbohydrates. It has higher levels of iron when compared to a similar serving size of beef, pork, lamb and chicken. It also contains higher potassium content with lower sodium levels, in other ways, it has more and other nutritional value with greater health benefits.

pig meat

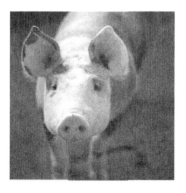

Pork is a great-tasting and good source of protein like poultry and is sometimes called white meat but is precisely red meat because it contains little myoglobin. It has almost the same nutrients as beef. It has less fat and calories, though this depends on the part you cut and prepare. It contains some important nutritional values such as protein, fat, saturated fat, sodium, and 0%carbohydrate, a 3-ounces portion of pig meat contain 239 calories if you eat both the slim and the fatty part. It also contains many of the micronutrients such as vitamins and minerals found in beef which help make and repair DNA and produce hormones and red blood cells and also a good source of vitamin B which its deficiencies can cause many problems in the mental health. Pork meat can be prepared and served in so many ways, such as pork sausage, pork bacon pulled pork Spam, all of this contains no carbohydrate unless prepared with barbecue sauce or some other sugar or starch.

Turkey meat

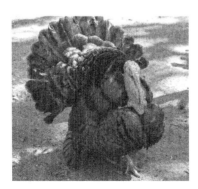

Turkey meat which is known as white meat and dark meat, the dark part is found in the legs or thighs, is rich in nutrients and a good source of protein and also has several important health benefits but the best is Pasture-raised or cage-free method of training, which exposes them to sunlight and a more various, natural diet that help in increasing their levels of nutrients such as omega-3 fatty acids Turkey is an excellent source of many vitamins and minerals such as Protein which is found vital for muscle growth and maintenance It gives structure to cells and helps transport nutrients around your body though a high protein diet can promote weight loss, it contains Fat, but mostly it comes from the skin , it contains 0% Carbohydrate, The B vitamins such as (Niacin) vitamin B3, Vitamin B6, Vitamin B12, these has many benefits and is important DNA production and the formation of red blood cells. Selenium is essential in the production of thyroid hormones, which normalize your metabolism and growth rate Zinc, which is important in bone health, Choline, and little of Magnesium and Potassium.

The 3-ounces portion of turkey meat contains 145 calories

Bacon

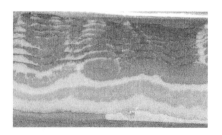

Bacon is made from the pork belly and back cuts, it is also made from other animals like turkey, but turkey bacon is slimmer than pork bacon. It usually comes in sliced, diced or spiral.

It contains 76% of fat, 25% protein 0% carbohydrate sodium, small cholesterol and a little iron.

The 3-ounces portion of bacon meat contains 390 calories.

Bison meat

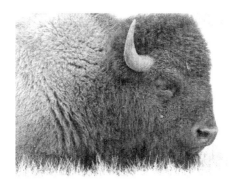

Bison has numerous essential nutrients, including protein, iron, zinc, selenium, and B vitamins, slightly low in calories, low in fat than many other types of meat and it also has less than 1-gram carbohydrate, which is not much. However, bison meat is considered an excellent source of protein and Sufficient protein intake is essential for numerous processes in your body, including tissue rebuilding, hormone production, and nutrient transport.

The 3-ounces portion of bison meat contains 190 calories.

Beef jerky

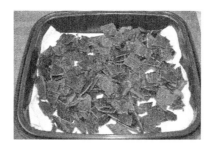

Beef jerky is always healthy and nutritious snack made from lean cuts of beef that are marinated with numerous spices, it's high in protein and low in carbs. It contains nutritional composition than other snakes, which makes it suitable for a low cab diet. It also contains various essential minerals and vitamins such as zinc, iron, vitamin B12, phosphorus, and folate. When it comes to snake food, beef jerky is always a good choice,

The 3-ounces portion of Beef jerky contain 349 calories.

Lamb meat

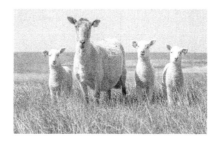

Lamb meat is a rich source of high-quality protein, and likewise, a source of many vitamins and minerals, including iron, zinc, selenium, healthy fat and as well an excellent

source of vitamin B12 and it contain 0% carb which makes it suitable for low cab diet

The 3-ounces portion of Lamb meat contains 176 calories.

Organ meat

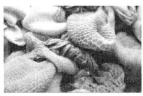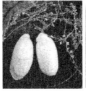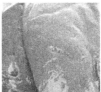

Organ meats are highly nutritional and excellent in protein fit for low cab diet, the organs include brains, liver, intestines and even testicles, they are considered more nutrient than muscle meat, but then the liver is most nutrient-dense than the other organ as it is a powerful source of vitamin A which is beneficial for eye health and for reducing diseases that cause inflammation, organ meat is rich in B-vitamins, such as vitamin B12 and folate, iron, magnesium, selenium, zinc, and vitamins A, D, E

The 3-ounces portion of brain 167, liver 115, testicles 106

Rabbit meat

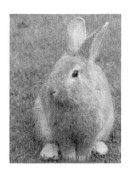

Rabbit meat is rich in nutrients and is a healthy source of animal protein. It has a very similar profile in vitamins close to those observed in chickens but has one of the lowest fat amounts in other consumed meat though the amount of fat in domestic and wild rabbits are substantially different, rabbits can easily be farmed because of their small size. However, the wild rabbit is often consumed, Wild rabbit and domesticated rabbit have some nutritional differences and are also considered to be fairly different in terms of the flavor, it contains essential minerals and vitamin and also 0% carbohydrate the 3-ounces portion of rabbit meat contains 175 calories.

Chapter 3

You are advised to choose oily fish and fresh over canned food.

Fish and shellfish as a low carb food

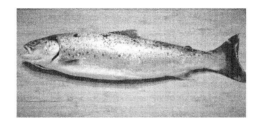

Fish is one of the healthiest foods on the planet, which include Cod, Tuna, Halibut, Mahi-mahi, Ocean perch, Salmon, Anchovies, lobster, mackerel, mussels, sardines, Tilapia, and many more. These have been an important source of protein and other nutrients, is much more than just a substitute source of animal protein. Fish is a good source of omega-3 fatty acids, which are extremely important for your

body, brain, eye health, and help to reduce the risk of heart disease. It also contains iodine, vitamin D, and various vitamins and minerals that people are lacking. If on a low carb diet or you're trying to lose weight or improve your diet, you should perhaps eat more fish and shellfish. Contains **0%** carbohydrate

The 3-ounces portion of oily fish contains 134 calories

Chapter 4

Best low carb Nut flours

Almond flour

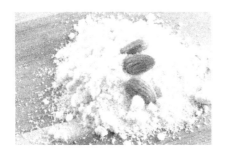

Almond flour is extremely nutritious and is one of the most popular low carb flours that might help stabilize blood sugar levels. Almond flour can be used for baking such as cakes, bread, and many others. The flour is high in protein more than the regular flour, it also contains manganese, vitamin E, monounsaturated fats, and fiber. The flour is suitable for those on gluten-free diets and low carb diet

56g of almond flour contains 324 calories

Total carb contains per 100 grams is 4.3g

Coconut flour

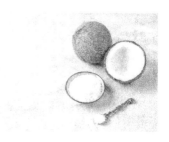

Coconut flour is highly beneficial when it comes to your health. It has a low content of carbohydrates compared to other nut flours, which makes it suitable for low carb diet, is considered a high protein content, low in calories, high in fiber, gluten-free and multipurpose when it comes to cooking and baking. Coconut flour contains the key vitamins and minerals which are essential in human such as manganese, calcium, and selenium. ½ cup of coconut flour contains 232 calories

Total carb contains per 100 grams is 76g

Psyllium Husk flour

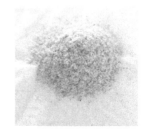

Psyllium husk is a type of dietary fiber that may help weight loss purposes, keto and low-carb baking, food industries frequently use psyllium to thicken bread products and cakes.

1tablespoon of Psyllium Husk flour contains 8 calories

Total carb contains per 100 grams is 80g

Chapter 5

Best low carb vegetables

Vegetables are low in calories, low in carbs and high in fiber, but rich in vitamins, minerals and other important nutrients. If you are on a low-carb lifestyle, the first thing that perhaps came to your mind is that you're going to eat a lot of vegetables to bulk up your meals rather than bread, pasta or rice. You can even have to eat as much as you want but then again, if on a low-carb diet or not eating more vegetables is always a great idea and a better choice when preparing meals. Although you also need to be aware of the carbs in vegetables, some vegetables such as starchy root vegetables should be avoided in large quantities. The best is the nonstarchy and green leafy vegetables. So, what vegetables are low in carbs? I've done the hard work for you. Below is the list of the best low carb vegetables and their carb percentage

Artichokes

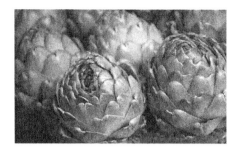

Total carb contains per 100 grams is 11g

100g of Artichokes contains 47 calories

Garden Asparagus

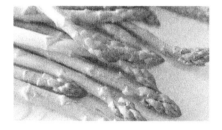

Total carb contains per 100 grams is 3.9g

100g of garden asparagus contains 20 calories

Aubergine

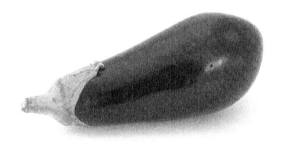

Total carb contains per 100 grams is 6g

100g of Aubergine contains 25 calories

Broccoli

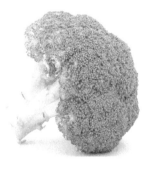

Total carb contains per 100 grams is 7g

100g of Broccoli contains 34 calories

Brussel sprouts

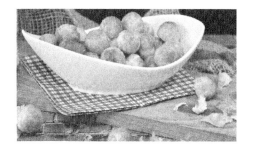

Total carb contains per 100 grams is 9g

100g of Brussel sprouts contains 43 calories

Cabbage

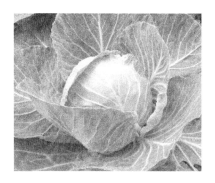

Total carb contains per 100 grams is 6g

100g of Cabbage contains 25 calories

Cauliflower

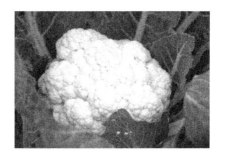

Total carb contains per 100 grams is 5g

100g of Cauliflower contains 25 calories

Celery

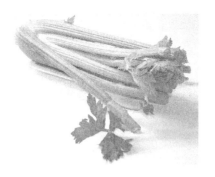

Total carb contains per 100 grams is 3g

100g of Celery contains 25 calories

Cucumber

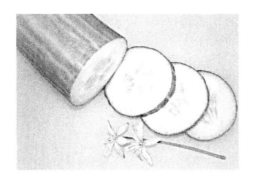

Total carb contains per 100 grams is 3.5g

100g of Cucumber contains 15 calories

Garlic

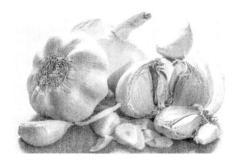

Total carb contains per 100 grams is 3.1g

100g of Garlic contains 149 calories

Green Beans

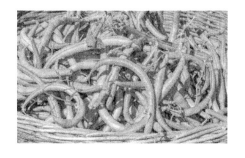

Total carb contains per 100 grams is 7g

100g of Green Beans contains 31 calories

Kale

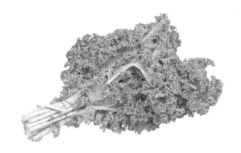

Total carb contains per 100 grams is 9g

100g of Kale contains 49 calories

Leeks

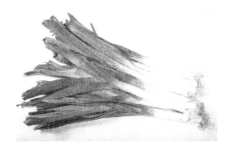

Total carb contains per 100 grams is 14g

100g of Leeks contains 61 calories

Mushrooms

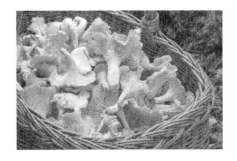

Total carb contains per 100 grams is 3.3g

100g of Mushrooms contains 22 calories

Okra

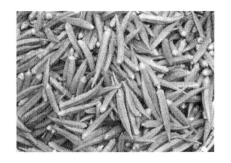

Total carb contains per 100 grams is 7g

100g of Okra contains 33 calories

Onions

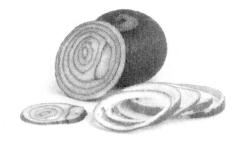

Total carb contains per 100 grams is 9g

100g of Onions contains 40 calories

Peppers

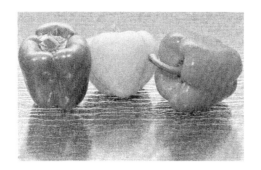

Total carb contains per 100 grams is 9g

100g of Peppers contains 40 calories

Pumpkin

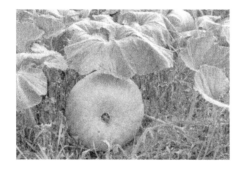

Total carb contains per 100 grams is 7g

100g of Pumpkin contains 26 calories

Radishes

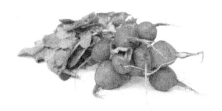

Total carb contains per 100 grams is 3.4g

100g of Radishes contains 16 calories

Spinach

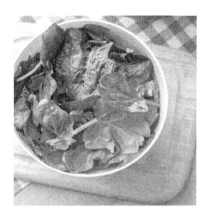

Total carb contains per 100 grams is 1.3g

100g of Spinach contains 16 calories

Sugar snap peas

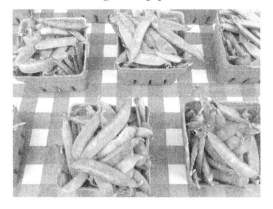

Total carb contains per 100 grams is 4.9g

100g of Sugar snap peas contains 34 calories

Tomatoes

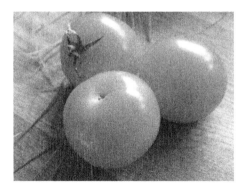

Total carb contains per 100 grams is 3.9g

100g of Tomatoes contains 18 calories

Zucchini

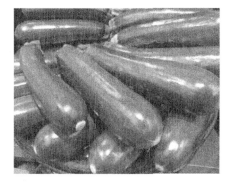

Total carb contains per 100 grams is 3.1g

100g of Zucchini contains 17 calories

Chapter 6

Best low carb fruits and berries

Fruits offer numerous important vitamins and nutrients that the body needs to function appropriately. Therefore, you don't have to remove them from your diet, even if you're on a low-carb diet, but some types of fruit can derail your low-carb diet. The key is to study which fruits are low in carbs and eat more of those. Fruits that are low in carbs offer nutritional benefits though still letting you stick to your low-carb diets. If you're trying to stick to a low-carb diet, below are great choices for you.

Peach

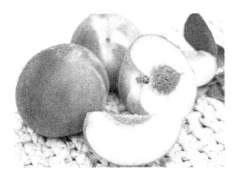

Peach is a good source of natural sugar, carbohydrate, vitamin A, vitamin C and little amount of fiber and protein

Total carb contains per 100 grams is 0 g

100g of Peach contains 39 calories

Rhubarb

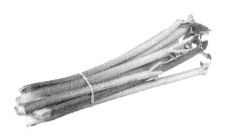

Rhubarb is an excellent source of vitamin C, vitamin K, potassium, and manganese and other lots of vitamins and minerals.

Total carb contains per 100 grams is 0g

100g of Rhubarb contains 21 calories

Clementine

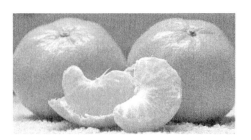

Clementine is rich in vitamin C and contain numerous other vitamins and minerals such as thiamine, folate, natural sugar and a small amount of protein

Total carb contains per 100 grams is 0 g

100g of Clementine contains 47 calories

Coconut

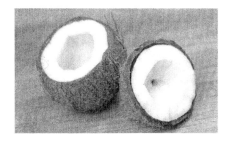

Coconut is high in saturated fat, and fiber. It also contains manganese, copper, selenium, phosphorus, potassium, and iron

Total carb contains per 100 grams is 3.7 g

100g of Coconut contains 354 calories

Olives

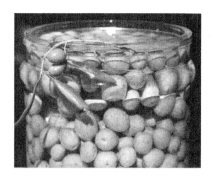

Olives are good source of a few micronutrients such as vitamin E, iron, copper and calcium

Total carb contains per 100 grams is 6.26 g

100g of Olives contains 145 calories

Strawberries

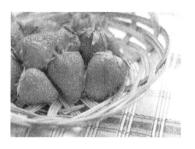

Strawberry is packed with vitamin C, manganese, fiber, antioxidants and also contain decent amounts of folate (vitamin B9), potassium and more

Total carb contains per 100 grams is 8 g

100g of Strawberries contains 33 calories

Cantaloupe

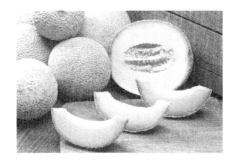

Cantaloupe contains the percent of the daily needs for vitamin C, fiber, vitamin A and is also a good source of potassium

Total carb contains per 100 grams is 8 g

100g of Cantaloupe contains 34 calories

Avocado

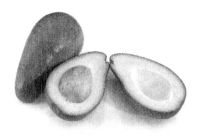

It contains fiber and are rich in vitamins and minerals, such as B-vitamins, vitamin K, potassium, copper, vitamin E, and vitamin C

Total carb contains per 100 grams is 9g

100g of Avocado contains 160 calories

Lemon

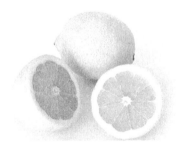

Lemon is a good source of vitamin C, folate, potassium and many more

Total carb contains per 100 grams is 9g

100g of Lemon contains 29 calories

Blackberries

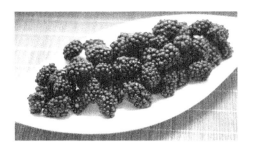

Blackberries is a good source of fiber, Vitamin E, Folate, Magnesium, Potassium, Copper, Vitamin C, Vitamin K and Manganese

Total carb contains per 100 grams is 10g

100g of Blackberries contains 43 calories

Lime

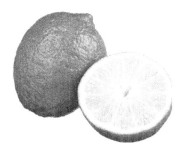

Limes are high in vitamin C and also contain small amounts of riboflavin, niacin, folate, phosphorus, magnesium iron, calcium, vitamin B6, thiamine, potassium, and more

Total carb contains per 100 grams is 11g

100g of Lime contains 30 calories

Raspberries

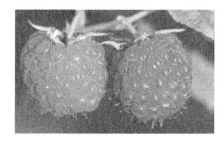

Raspberries is a good source of fiber, vitamin C Vitamin A, thiamine, riboflavin, vitamin B6, calcium and zinc

Total carb contains per 100 grams is 12g

100g of Raspberries contains 53 calories

Cherries

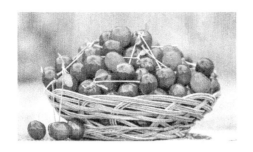

Cherries contains vital nutrients such as the B vitamins, manganese, copper, magnesium, vitamin K, vitamin C, potassium, and fiber,

Total carb contains per 100 grams is 12g

100g of Cherries contains 50 calories

Blueberries

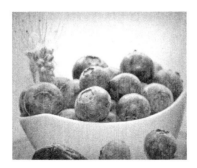

Blueberries is high in fiber, contains vitamin C and vitamin K and several important nutrients.

Total carb contains per 100 grams is 14g

100g of Blueberries contains 57 calories

Kiwi

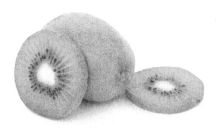

Kiwis has a good health benefits and full of nutrients such as vitamin C, vitamin K, vitamin E, folate, fiber, antioxidants and potassium.

Total carb contains per 100 grams is 15g

100g of Kiwi contains 61 calories

Chapter 7

Best low carb drinks

In a low carb diet, what you eat matters, and so does what you drink. Many drinks contain carbs that can derail your low-carb diet, although Keeping well hydrated is important to feel good. Below is a list of drinks and the number of grams of carbs per 100gram

Coffee

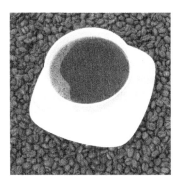

Coffee is an excellent source of antioxidants and also contains an immune-boosting natural nutrient

Total carb contains per 100 grams is 0g

100g of Coffee contains 0 calories

All teas without adding sugar or milk

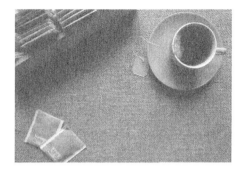

Tea is a beverage made from a common dried tea plant, and it contains a whole lot of health benefits so also an antioxidant property. Its fermentation determines the color of the tea, which might be white, green, or black in colour. It is commonly prepared by pouring hot or boiling water over dried or fresh leaves in a cup for 1 to 5 minutes

Total carb contains per 100 grams is 0.2g

100g of Tea contains 1 calorie

Lemon juice

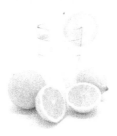

Lemon juice has many important health benefits, and is also a good source of vitamin B6, vitamin C, folate, potassium, fiber, antioxidants and several other vitamins and minerals

Total carb contains per 100 grams is 9g

100g of Lemon juice contains 22 calories

Lime juice

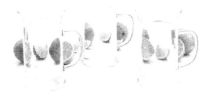

Limes are high in vitamin C and also contain small amounts of riboflavin, niacin, folate, phosphorus, magnesium iron, calcium, vitamin B6, thiamine, potassium, and more

Total carb contains per 100 grams is 8g

100g of Lime juice contains 0 calories

Water

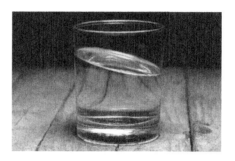

Water is perfect when it is transparent, tasteless, odorless, and nearly colorless. It is a great thirst-quencher. even though it provides no organic nutrients and it has no carbs

Total carb contains per 100 grams is 0g

100g of Water contains 0 calories

Chapter 8

Low carb Nuts & Seeds

Almonds

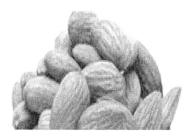

Almonds are highly nutritious edible seeds, rich in healthy fats, antioxidants, vitamins and minerals. They are low in carbs but high in healthy fats, protein, fiber and various important nutrients.

Total carb contains per 100 grams is 13.3g

100g of almond contains 607 calories

Brazil Nuts

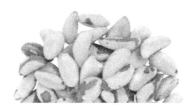

Brazil nuts are one of the richest dietary sources of selenium, an essential mineral with antioxidant and anti-inflammatory properties, as well as being a good source of important nutrients including zinc, magnesium, fiber, calcium, vitamin E and some B vitamins. It also has a high proportion of monounsaturated fat, which is a good fat, and some protein

Total carb contains per 100 grams is 12g

100g of Brazil Nuts contains 700 calories

Macadamia Nuts

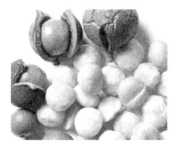

Macadamia nuts are high in healthy fats, vitamins, minerals and may help those trying to lose weight. It also contains

antioxidants protein, manganese, dietary fiber, thiamin, and copper. Eating small amounts each day may help reduce cardiovascular disease risk factors

Total carb contains per 100 grams is 14g

100g of Macadamia Nuts contains 718 calories

Pine nuts

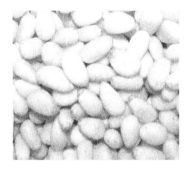

Pine nuts are rich in monounsaturated fatty acids, high in vitamins such as vitamin E, vitamin K, vitamin B-6 and antioxidants, which helps in preventing coronary artery disease and its potential use in weight loss. Moreover, it also contains healthy amounts of essential minerals such as magnesium, iron, zinc, calcium, phosphorus, manganese, potassium and selenium

Total carb contains per 100 grams is 13g

100g of pine nuts contains 673 calories

Hazelnuts

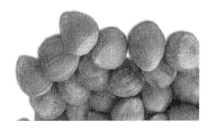

Hazelnuts are a rich source of mono- and polyunsaturated fats and likewise omega-6 and omega-9 fatty acids. The nuts are loaded with dietary fiber, vitamins, and minerals and extremely rich in folate. In sum, they help protect from diseases and cancers

Total carb contains per 100 grams is 17g

100g of Hazelnuts contains 628 calories

Walnuts

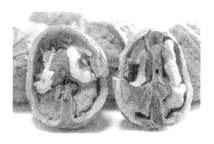

Walnuts are an excellent source of numerous vitamins and minerals. These comprise copper, folic acid, phosphorus, vitamin B6, manganese, vitamin and smaller amounts of iron, calcium, zinc, potassium, and selenium. They are a good source of protein and fiber, making them a smart food for weight loss

Total carb contains per 100 grams is 14g

100g of Walnuts contains 654 calories

Flaxseed

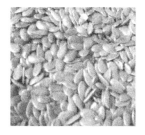

Flaxseeds contain high fiber that can help lower cholesterol, as well as protein, omega-3 fatty acids which are present in fish, some vitamins and minerals along with phytochemicals called lignans

Total carb contains per 100 grams is 28g

100g of flaxseed contains 534 calories

Hemp seed

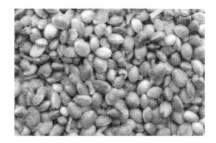

Hemp seed is rich in fatty-acid profile, which includes omega-3 and -6 fatty acids. It is also a great source of protein and calcium, and other essential vitamins and minerals, plus less common stearidonic (SDA) and gamma linoleic (GLA) acids. Hemp seed testes pretty good

Total carb contains per 100 grams is 6.58g

100g of hemp seed contains 566 calories

Pumpkin seed

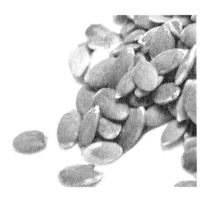

Pumpkin seeds are highly nutritious and packed with zinc, magnesium, potassium, vitamin B2 (riboflavin), folate, fatty acids, dietary fiber, and powerful antioxidants. They also contain a good series of nutrients as well as iron, selenium and calcium

Total carb contains per 100 grams is 54g

100g of pumpkin seed contains 446 calories

Chia seed

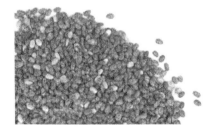

Chia seeds are one of the healthiest foods on earth. They're loaded with nutrients that are beneficial to our body and brain. They contain omega-3 fatty acids, rich in antioxidants, and they provide fiber, iron, magnesium, phosphorus protein and calcium and some other decent amount of zinc, vitamin

B3 (niacin), potassium, vitamin B1 (thiamine) and vitamin B2. Chia seeds can be consumed cooked or raw, but they should be added as a supplement to another food

Total carb contains per 100 grams is 42g

100g of chia seed contains 486 calories

Sunflower seeds

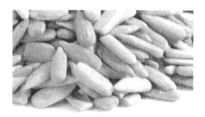

Sunflower seeds are pretty rich in B complex vitamins, which are important for a healthy nervous system. They are an excellent source of phosphorus, magnesium, iron, calcium, potassium, protein and vitamin E. They also a good natural

source of minerals, zinc, manganese, copper, chromium and carotene, as well as monounsaturated and polyunsaturated fatty acids.

Total carb contains per 100 grams is 20g

100g of sunflower seed contains 584 calories

Chapter 9

The best Alcohol to be taken when on low carb diet

Brandy

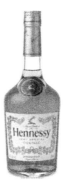

Total carb contains per 100 grams is 0g

100g of Brandy contains 231calories

Gin

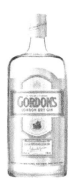

Total carb contains per 100 grams is 0g

100g of Gin contains 263 calories

Vodka

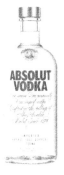

Total carb contains per 100 grams is 0g

100g of vodka contains 231 calories

Whiskey

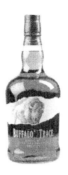

Total carb contains per 100 grams is 0g

100g of whiskey contains 250 calories

Tequila

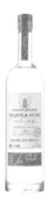

Total carb contains per 100 grams is 0g

100g of Tequila contains 231 calories

Chapter 10

Low carb dairy

You are advised to avoid low-fat and fat-free dairy

Eggs

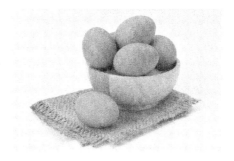

Eggs are among the most healthful foods that contain a fairly low-calorie and a very small amount of carbohydrate 0.6g. Furthermore, an egg is an excellent source of protein and contain various important nutrients, which include vitamins A, B, E, K, D, zinc, calcium, and many more

The 3-ounces portion of Egg contains 125 calories.

Butter

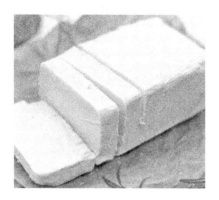

Total carb contains per 100 grams is 0.1g

100g of Butter contains 717 calories

Ghee

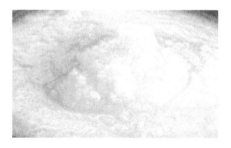

Total carb contains per 100 grams is 0g

100g of Ghee contains 849 calories

Cheese

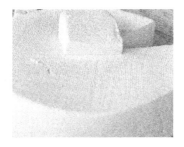

Total carb contains per 100 grams is 0g

100g of Cheese contains 402 calories

Yogurt

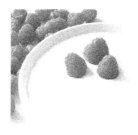

Total carb contains per 100 grams is 3.6g

100g of Yogurt contains 59 calories

Chapter 11

Best low carb fats

Olive oil

Total carb contains per 100 grams is 0g

100g of Olive oil contains 884 calories

Ghee

Total carb contains per 100 grams is 0g

100g of Ghee contains 849 calories

Goose fat

Total carb contains per 100 grams is 0g

100g of Goose fat contains 900 calories

Lard

Total carb contains per 100 grams is 0g

100g of Lard contains 898 calories

Macadamia oil

Total carb contains per 100 grams is 0g

100g of Macadamia oil contains 718 calories

Mayonnaise

Total carb contains per 100 grams is 9.23g

100g of Mayonnaise contains 680 calories

Avocado oil

Total carb contains per 100 grams is 0g

100g of Avocado oil contains 884 calories

Butter

Total carb contains per 100 grams is 0g

100g of Butter contains 717 calories

Cocoa butter

Total carb contains per 100 grams is 0g

100g of Cocoa butter contains 884 calories

Coconut oil

Total carb contains per 100 grams is 0g

100g of Coconut oil contains 862 calories

Duck fat

Total carb contains per 100 grams is 0g

100g of Duck fat contains 882 calories

Chapter 12

7 days easy to follow low carb nutritional plan

MONDAY

BREAKFAST: Scrambled Eggs & Bacon

INGREDIENT: 5 large eggs, 7 slices bacon, salt to test, 1/8 tsp pepper, 2 tbs of butter, 2tbs chopped leeks.

METHOD: Cook the bacon till crisp by adding a little water in a saucepan, then allow water to dry off on the fire or remove from pan drain the bacon on paper towels and reserve, in a large bowl, beat the eggs with salt and pepper, return the saucepan to medium heat and add the butter, melt butter over medium heat, then add the beaten eggs over medium heat, infrequently stirring with a heat-proof spatula, scraping to form large curds until the eggs are almost set., pour the reserved bacon and stir continue cooking till eggs are set, then garnish with the leeks, serve hot and enjoy

LUNCH: chicken salad

3 cups of mashed cooked chicken

2 cloves of chopped Garlic

1/4 cup Mayonnaise

2 fresh chopped tomatoes

½ cup of chopped onions

½ cup of chopped cabbage

Sea salt to test

Black pepper

Procedure

Stir together the mayonnaise, onions, tomatoes, fresh cabbage, and garlic until smooth.

Stir in the chicken and season with sea salt and black pepper to taste. Then your super easy chicken salad is ready.

SNACK: Beef jerky

DINNER: Grilled chicken with vegetables.

6 chicken breasts

1 tbs lemon juice

1 tsp of garlic powder

1 tsp of dried rosemary

½ tsp sea salt

½ tsp black pepper

½ tsp onion powder

1/3 cup mayonnaise

Procedure

Combine the seasonings, divide the sauce into two. Brush the chicken with half of the sauce and let marinate in the refrigerator for at least 2 and up to 6 hours, preheat a grill and grill a medium-high heat, then cover the grill for 7 minutes, flip and brush with the reserved marinade. Grill for about 7 minutes more, until the meat is ready

Tuesday

BREAKFAST: Omelette with mushrooms

4 eggs

4 mushrooms sliced

1 oz butter

¼ onion chopped

Sea salt

½ black pepper

procedure

Crack the eggs into a bowl, then add a pinch of salt and pepper. Whisk the eggs with a fork until smooth and foamy, dissolve the butter in a frying pan over medium heat, add the mushrooms and onion to the pan, stirring until tender, and then gently pour in the egg mixture surrounding the veggies.

When the omelet begins to cook and get firm, using a frying spatula, carefully ease around the edges of the omelet, and then fold it over in half. Then remove from the pan and place on the plate when it starts to turn golden brown under

LUNCH: Grass-fed yogurt with berries, coconut flakes and walnuts

8 oz. grass-fed yogurt

1/2 cup blueberries

1 tbsp. unsweetened coconut flakes

A handful of walnuts, chopped

Procedure

Get a bowl, pour in the yogurt and place the rest of the ingredients on top

SNACK: macadamia nuts

DINNER: Pork chops with vegetables

3/4-pound pork chops

4 tbs olive oil (divided)

1 tbs chopped fresh ginger

1 tsp pounded garlic

12 ounces broccoli florets

1 red bell pepper, chopped into strips

1 bunch green onions chopped

4 tbsp Dijon mustard

1/2 tsp sea salt, or to taste

1/4 tsp pepper, or to taste

2 tbsp minced rosemary and thyme

Procedure

In a skillet, put the chopped ginger, garlic and pork and mix with 1tbs of oil and set separate, place the bell pepper into the bottom of a medium bowl then add the green onions and cut the broccoli florets into large bite sized pieces, layering them on top in a separate bowl and set aside mix the rest of the ingredient in a bowl with little water and add to the skillet. Then Place over high heat. It's ready when a drop of water hops across the surface. Add 1 tablespoon of oil and quickly tilt the work to coat all surfaces. Pour out the remaining oil. Place the food back on the heat and allow the pork until it has cooked halfway to turn white. Stir the pork and cook until it is almost tender. Remove from the pan and place the bowl of vegetables into a pan with the broccoli in the bottom. Cover with the lid of the skillet and cook for 1 minute. Stir the vegetables and add the prepared pork and any juices back to the pan. Stir the pork and vegetables together, then Pour the sauce over the stir fry when it reaches your desired level of thickness

Or you can use another technique of your choice

Wednesday

BREAKFAST: Cauliflower Hash Brown Egg Cups

Preparation and cook time: 55 minutes

Serving 12

A medium-size of cauliflower, (cut into flowerets and steamed)

2 cups of shredded cheddar

14 large eggs (divided)

1 tbs of blended garlic

1 tsp of salt

3 slices of cooked bacon (smashed)

Chives (sliced)

Black pepper (pounded)

Procedures

Heat oven to 375° and set aside a lightly grease 12-cup muffin tin using butter or oil then Place steamed cauliflower in a food processor and blend until it forms a fine grain, at that moment remove and pour into paper towels and twist to remove the water completely leaving the cauliflower dry. In a big bowl, put together the dry cauliflower, cheddar, garlic, 2 eggs, and salt to test then pour the mixture evenly between 12 muffin tins, ensure each tin contains about ¼ of the mixture., with your fingers press the mixture inside the tins to form nests, place in an oven and bake for about 15 to 17 minutes until the edges change to golden, then remove from oven and Sprinkle bacon to the bottom of each tin, crash an egg on top of each bacon and make sure that the yolk remains intact, then put the tins back inside the oven and bake for about 7 to 8 minutes until the egg becomes sets, remove from oven and sprinkle with pepper and chives, the food is ready

LUNCH: Chicken Curry

Preparation and cook time: 45 minutes

Servings 6

2 pounds of skinless chicken breasts (slice into pieces)

2 to 3 tablespoon of extra-virgin olive oil

1 medium yellow onion (sliced)

3 cloves garlic crushed

1 tablespoon crushed ginger

1½ tsp paprika

1½ tsp pounded turmeric

1½ tsp of pounded coriander

1 tsp of pounded cumin

1 can or 15-oz crushed tomatoes

1½ cups of low-sodium chicken broth

1/2 cup of heavy cream

Acceptable salt for taste

1 tsp of freshly crushed black pepper

Basmati rice for serving

1 tablespoon freshly chopped cilantro (garnish)

Procedures

Put oil in a large pot and place over a medium heat, stir in onion and cook until it becomes soft then pour the chicken into the pot and cook for about 5 minutes or, until the pink color goes, add ginger and garlic and stir-fry for a minute or until fragrant, add up the remaining spices in the ingredients section and cook for about a minute, at that point add the broth and tomatoes and bring it to a simmer, add heavy whipping cream and season with pepper and salt to taste, Cook the chicken for about 15 to 20 minutes or until chicken bits become tender.

Serve over rice and garnished with cilantro.

SNACK: Avocado

DINNER: Grilled chicken wings with spinach on the side.

6 chicken wings

1 tbs lemon juice

1 tsp of garlic powder

1 tsp of dried rosemary

½ tsp sea salt

½ tsp black pepper

½ tsp onion powder

1/3 cup mayonnaise

Procedure

Combine the seasonings, divide the sauce into two. brush the chicken with half of the sauce and let marinade in the refrigerator for at least 2 and up to 6 hours, preheat a grill and grill a medium high heat, then cover the grill for 7 minutes, flip and brush with the reserved marinate. Grill for about 7 minutes more, until the meat is ready, then slice the spinach by the side and enjoy.

Thursday

BREAKFAST: Baked Avocado Eggs

Preparation 30 minutes

Serving: 4

2 Medium-size ripe avocados

4 large eggs

Salt to taste

Pepper to taste

1/4 cup or 55g bacon bits

1 cherry tomato (cut into four)

1 spring of fresh basil sliced

A handful of shredded cheddar cheese

2 tablespoons of fresh chives (sliced)

Procedures

Cut and open the avocados into two to remove the seeds then with a spoon, scoop out some of the flesh to create a bigger hole and place the halves of the avocado on a baking sheet, at that moment preheat and set oven to 400°F or 200°C, in each of the holes, crack one egg inside and make sure the yolk remains intact, Season with pepper and salt, add fresh basil, tomatoes, bacon, cheddar cheese, and chives, put the baking sheet in an oven and bake for about 15 minutes then remove from the oven and serve

LUNCH: Ground beef zucchini with pesto

Preparation and cook time: 20 minutes

Servings 6

1 lb. of Ground beef

1 tsp of Sea salt

1/2 tsp of Black pepper

2 medium sizes of Zucchini (cut in shape of half-moons)

2 cloves of Garlic (crushed)

3/4 cup Basil pesto

1/2 cup crumbled Goat cheese

2 tablespoon of fresh parsley (sliced)

Procedures

On a large skillet over medium heat, add garlic and stir-fry until fragrant, add ground beef then stir in salt and ground pepper to taste bring up the heat to high and allow to cook for 7 to 10 minutes break part with a spoon infrequently as you stir until browned, stir in zucchini and cook for 5-7 minutes, stir infrequently until it starts to get soft and become golden, bring down from heat and stir in basil pesto, garnish with fresh parsley and goat cheese, ready to serve

SNACK: Strawberries & cream

DINNER: Chicken Breasts with Mushroom and Cream Sauce

Servings: 4

4 chicken breasts (with the skin and bone removed)

2 cups of sliced mushrooms

1/2 cup onions (cut up)

2 tbs of flour

3/4 cup milk

3 tbs olive oil

2 tbs fresh thyme leaves (sliced)

1 clove of garlic (crushed)

1/4 tsp sea salt for taste

1/4 tsp black pepper

Procedures

Season the smashed chicken breasts with salt and pepper and place aside, place a skillet pan over medium heat and add one tablespoon of olive oil, add the chicken breasts then cook for 1 minute until the color become golden on the bottom, then turn over and reduce the heat, cover the pan with a lid, cook the chicken for 10 minutes without removing the lid., still with the lid intact after 10 minutes, remove the skillet from the heat, leave it for extra 10 minutes, this is to make sure that the chicken breast is cooked well, remove the chicken from the pan, cover to stay warm and set aside.

Place another empty pan over medium heat and add one tablespoon of olive oil then Stir in onions and mushrooms and allow to cook for about 5 to 8 minutes or until the mushrooms releases water and the water evaporates, add two tablespoon flour and cook for extra 2 minutes until fragrant, stir in garlic and cook for 30 seconds, stir in thyme, 1/4 milk, salt and pepper, turn until the mixture becomes thick, pour another 1/4 cup of milk and turn until everything thickened, on a serving plate, place the chicken and pour the sauce over it, ready to serve and enjoy

Friday

BREAKFAST: mixed Cereal

Preparation: 35 minutes

Serving 4

1/4 cup sesame seeds

1 cup of chopped almonds

1 cup of chopped walnuts

1 cup of unsweetened coconut flakes

2 tbs of flax seeds

2 tbs of chia seeds

1/2 tsp of crushed clove

1½ tsp of powdered cinnamon

1 tsp of pure vanilla extract

½ tsp of kosher salt

1 large egg white

1/4 cup of liquefied coconut oil

Procedures

Heat up oven to 350°, Lubricant the baking sheet with cooking spray, then in a large bowl, add walnuts, almonds, coconut flakes, flax seeds, sesame seeds, and chia seeds, and mix thoroughly to combine, stir in cloves, vanilla, cinnamon, and salt, in another separate bowl, whisk the egg white until it becomes foamy and stir the egg white into the cereal, stir in coconut oil and mix very well, pour and spread the mixture evenly onto the prepared baking sheet, place inside an oven and allow it to bake for 20 to 25 minutes, or until it becomes golden in color, remember to stir at an interval, remove from oven and allow it to cool completely, food is ready to Serve and enjoy

LUNCH Baked cauliflower and cheese

Preparation: 25 minutes

Servings 4

1 medium head of Cauliflower (cut into small buds)

3 tbs of butter

kosher salt for taste

1 tsp of Black pepper

1 cup cheddar cheese (shredded)

1/4 cup of Heavy cream

1/4 cup of unsweetened almond milk (or any milk of choice)

Procedures

Heat up the oven to 450 degrees F

In a baking sheet, line with foil or parchment paper, in a large bowl, combine cauliflower florets and 2 tbs of melted butter then mix properly. Season the mixture with salt and pepper to test, then arrange the cauliflower florets in the already prepared baking sheet and place in an oven and allow it to roast for about 10-15 minutes or until crisp-tender, remove from the oven and set aside.

At that point

In a clean skillet place over medium heat, add cheddar cheese, milk, heavy cream, 1 tablespoon of butter and stir frequently to prevent burning, allow to heat until the cheese mixture becomes smooth; make sure the cheese.is not burnt then remove from heat and pour the cheese mixture over the cauliflower, ready to serve and enjoy

SNACK Hardboiled egg

DINNER. One cup of plain yogurt: With chopped almonds or walnuts and ground flax seed

Saturday

BREAKFAST: Omelette with fresh tomatoes and mushroom

4 eggs

4 mushrooms sliced

2 fresh tomatoes sliced

1 oz butter

¼ onion chopped

Sea salt

½ black pepper

procedure

Crack the eggs into a bowl and then add a pinch of salt and pepper. Whisk the eggs with a fork until smooth and foamy, dissolve the butter in a frying pan, over medium heat, add the mushrooms, tomatoes and onion to the pan, stirring until tender, and then gently pour in the egg mixture surrounding the veggies, when the omelette begins to cook and get firm, using a frying spatula, carefully use the spatula to ease around the edges of the omelette in the frying pan, and then fold it over in half. Then remove from the pan and place on the plate when it starts to turn golden brown under

LUNCH: Turkey chili

1 pound of ground turkey

2 fresh tomatoes diced

Cinnamon powder

Chili powder

½ green pepper diced

2 tbs of olive oil

1 ball of onion

Sea salt to test

Procedure

Put the oil in a non-stick skillet and place over a medium heat, pour the turkey and stir till is brown then transfer to a plate, add oil to the skillet and stir in the vegetables (tomato, onion, green pepper), cinnamon chili and salt to test cook till tender the pour in the turkey mix thoroughly and remove from heat, your meal is ready

SNACK: 2 fresh cucumber sliced

DINNER: Chicken & green vegetables

Time: 22 minutes

Serving :4

2 Tbs coconut oil

1 lb chicken breasts

Sea salt for test

pepper

1 Tbs herbs de Provence (sub Tuscan Seasoning)

8 oz green beans, (trimmed)

8 oz asparagus, (woody ends removed)

2 garlic cloves, (minced)

½ Cup cherry tomatoes, halved

procedure

Season the chicken with herbs de Provence, salt and pepper then put the chicken to the skillet and cook, until fully cooked, remove chicken from skillet, and keep warm. Heat oil in a large skillet over medium high heat, add green vegetables (green beans, asparagus) and cook until tender, then add garlic and cook about 30 seconds, then add the tomatoes and season with salt and pepper, pour the cooked veggies into plates, and top with chicken.

Sunday

BREAKFAST: scrambled eggs & bacon

LUNCH: avocado and diced cooked pork, mixed thoroughly

SNACK: almond nut

DINNER: Easy and fast avocado mash

Time: 40 minutes

2 medium-size avocados

1 small onion (finely sliced)

1 clove of garlic (pounded)

1 ripe medium tomato (sliced)

1 small size lime (juiced)

Sea salt for test

1/2 teaspoon of pepper

Procedures

Cut the avocado into two, remove the seed and skin and then put the flesh into a medium bowl and Mash with a spatula, stir in garlic, onions, lime juice, tomato, salt, and pepper., adjust the seasoning where necessary, then put the bowl containing avocado in a fridge for an hour to blend the flavor, remove and serve

Printed in Great Britain
by Amazon